— What Student

"I was finally able to hook my fingers together in the Gomukasana..."

And here is why I'm so happy today... I've been taking the YOGABODY supplements and doing the Gravity stretches for about two months now. I've been noticing improvements along the way, like being able to put my hands on the ground above my head when I lie on my back. And my back bends are going places they've never been before. But today, I was finally able to hook my fingers together in the Gomukasana arms on both sides. Thanks Lucas!

- Jason Alan Griffin (Nia Teacher & Personal Trainer)

"I can feel a huge difference!"

Thank you for all of your mails and for The YOGABODY Handbook... the Gravity Poses are amazing! After just two days of doing them, I can feel a huge difference! Can't wait for day three today...

- Vesna Bacic (Yoga Student)

"I am sleeping much better..."

The supplements combined with your Gravity Poses seem to be working... I easily held full front splits for five minutes (both sides) the other day—haven't done that for a while! I have also noticed that I am sleeping much better. I don't know whether it is the extra stretching or eating more fruit and vegetables that has improved my sleep, maybe it's both.

- Iain Campbell (Yoga Student)

"I can put my hands FLAT ON THE FLOOR!!!!"

Lucas, I had to share an amazing thing I discovered this morning: When I bend at my waist and keep my legs straight, I can put my hands FLAT ON THE FLOOR! You gotta understand how cool this is—I am 40 years old, and I have NEVER been able to do that in my entire LIFE! When I started YOGABODY six weeks ago, I couldn't even touch my TOES! Thank you thank you thank you thank you. This is incredible!

- Margie Remmers (Yoga Student)

"Able to sit in lotus pose for about 1 hour now..."

I have been using your Gravity Poses to loosen my hips and they have done wonders. I have been able to sit in lotus pose for about 1 hour now without tremendous discomfort.

- Stephen McConnell (Yoga Student)

"I love how I feel..."

I love how I feel now that I have stepped up my practice and am using the Gravity Poses and YOGABODY.

- James Oddie (Yoga Student)

"I feel more focused and balanced."

I am just on my second day... and like the many people whom you have helped, I too notice a difference. I'm not as tired, and I feel more focused and balanced. I know that there is more to expect from YOGABODY so I am excited by all the discoveries still to be had on my mat during practice. Thank you so much for being so generous with what you have learned and sharing it with people who just want to deepen their practice. May you receive a hundred fold all that you so willingly give to people.

- Delamar Arias (Yoga Student)

"Lighter, stronger and I'm gaining in flexibility every day!"

I'm a yoga teacher in Milan, Italy. I started to take your tablets one week ago, and I'm on your Gravity Poses right now. It works!! I really feel lighter, stronger and I'm gaining in flexibility every day!! Thank you so much. I also like to read your tips in the newsletter. Simple little things but very effective!

- Ingrid Pistolesi (Yoga Teacher)

"They really work..."

I'm practicing the stretching exercises you sent me and they really work. The movement in my hips has improved a lot, which is my primary concern... Keep practicing!

- Milagros Capriles (Yoga Student)

"YOGABODY rocks!"

I am on day 25 of what was to be a 30-day challenge which now I have decided to go for 60 days straight. The recovery is so much quicker and with the additional stretching I feel like my Bikram has improved 100%—many, many thanks!

- Juliann Schuett (Yoga Student)

THE YOGABODY HANDBOOK

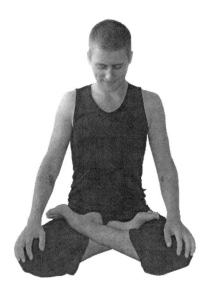

The Definitive Guide to Maximum
Flexibility (in Just 15 Minutes Per Day)

By Lucas Rockwood

Registered Yoga Teacher (E-RYT 200) & Nutritional Coach

THE YOGABODY HANDBOOK

ISBN: 978-0-9844328-0-6 Copyright © 2010
by Lucas Rockwood

Published by
YOGABODY Naturals Publishing

This publication is designed to provide accurate and authoritative information on yoga and nutrition. It is sold with the understanding that neither the publisher nor the author is engaged in providing medical advice. Before beginning any new exercise or diet regime, it's always wise to consult with your health care provider.

Find us online:

www.YogaBodyNaturals.com

www.YogaProtein.com

www.TheYogaTrapeze.com

www.YogaOmega3.com

www.YogaB12.com

www.YogaDeepSleep.com

www.MyYogaBusiness.com

ART & REFERENCES: Quotations throughout this book are from teachers I have met, read, or watched who have inspired me. The photos included (that are not me) are of people who are better looking than me.

CONTENTS

Preface .... pg. 11

Anthony's Three Flexibility Secrets .... pg. 15

Myth vs. Reality .... pg. 17

Improving Flexibility .... pg. 21

Food & Flexibility .... pg. 25

Flexibility Superfoods... pg.29

Drink More Water. .... pg. 33

The Bad Foods .... pg. 37

The YOGABODY Diet .... pg. 41

Nutritional Supplements. .... pg. 49

Where Do You Get Your Protein? .... pg. 53

What About Vitamin B12?.. pg. 57

Do I Need to Eat Fish? .... pg. 59

How to Stretch .... pg. 63

Gravity Poses.. pg. 65

Stretching Tips .... pg. 69

Stretching Schedule .... pg. 73

Complete Gravity Pose Chart..................................... pg. 76

Day 1: Hamstrings.. pg. 79

Day 2: Hips .... pg. 83

Day 3: Shoulders.. pg. 87

Day 4: Back .... pg. 91

Day 5: Wrists, Twists & Ankles................................... pg. 97

Frequent Questions .... pg. 103

About the Author .... pg. 109

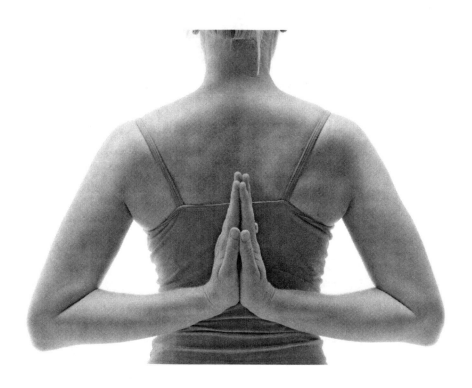

"Blessed are the flexible, for they shall
not be bent out of shape."
~ *Anonymous*

PREFACE

At the end of 8th grade, my entire school was forced to take a "stretch test" during physical education class. When it was my turn, I sat down and attempted to reach for my toes in a forward fold while the teacher measured my flexibility with a ruler.

The other kids huddled around with anticipation waiting to see how far I could stretch, but with my hands just halfway down my shins (still a good 8 inches shy of my toes), I'd already reached my limit!

"Go on, Luke, stretch!" the teacher said, so I gritted my teeth and bounced and bounced and bounced, but it was hopeless! My classmates began to snicker, and the teacher thought I was being a smartass.

"Try again," she said, and I closed my eyes and thrust my body forward until my hamstrings screamed. I figured that I'd at least reached my toes, but when I opened my eyes, I was still 6 inches away! That was it. The moment of truth.

For the first time in my life, I realized that my body was completely stiff and inflexible. And with all my classmates laughing, I made a public announcement that went something like this:

"Stretching is stupid, painful, and a complete waste of time!" Irony in action: fast forward 10 years to New York City, to my first yoga class.

My hips were so tight that I couldn't squat down, and my wrists and ankles were so locked up that I couldn't hold down dog for more than a few breaths. While I knew that yoga was good for me, I still HATED stretching. My body felt impossibly stiff, and I knew that traditional yoga and stretching exercises weren't going to cut it... and then I met a guy named, Anthony, at Bikram Yoga Soho in New York City who completely changed my life.

Anthony was not your average yoga guy. He lived with his mom in the East Village and he'd spent the last two years extremely ill with a bizarre nerve condition that no doctor could effectively treat.

But here's one thing I know for sure: when you're sick, tired, worn-down, out of shape, and so stiff that it hurts to bring your arms up over your head—that's when you start looking for solutions.

Since yoga reduced Anthony's nerve pain right away, he started practicing every day. Anthony was carrying extra weight, just like me, and he was stiff—really stiff! We were nearly identical in build, and since we usually practiced side-by-side, it was impossible not to compare our progress.

But here's the thing: Anthony was putting me to shame!

He lost weight quickly and was getting strong AND flexible fast, while I was lucky to make it through the standing postures without getting queasy. In yoga, you're supposed to stay focused, but I couldn't help staring.

After 6 weeks, Anthony could lie flat against his thighs in forward bends, cross his legs in full lotus, and drop back three times deeper in backbends than I could. I wasn't just jealous—I was pissed off!

"What's this guy doing that I'm not doing?"

So one night after class, I invited Anthony for pizza (this was before I became vegan), and although Anthony didn't eat a thing, ***he did tell me three secrets to stretching flexibility that I later learned are 100% true for everyone.***

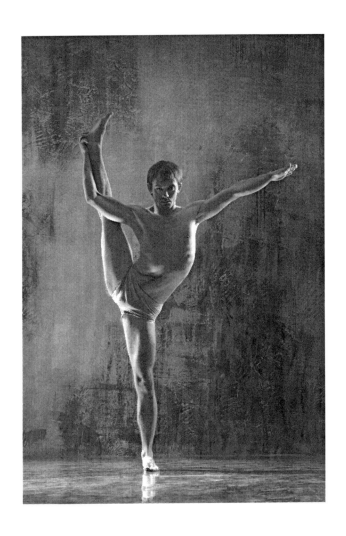

"When you inhale, you are taking the strength from God. When you exhale, it represents the service you are giving to the world."
~ B.K.S. Iyengar

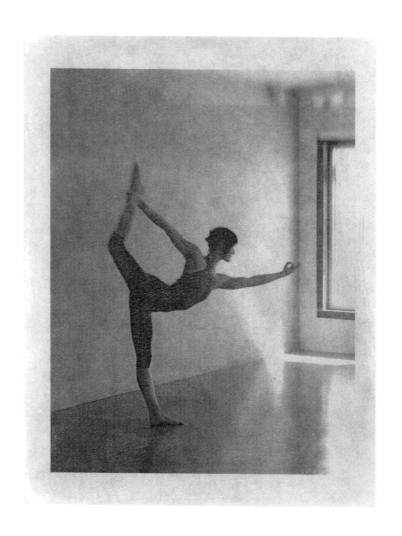

"Your vision will become clear only when you look into your heart... he who looks *outside*, dreams. He who looks *inside*, awakens."
~ *Carl Jung*

ANTHONY'S THREE FLEXIBILITY SECRETS

1. ANYONE CAN BECOME FLEXIBLE

Guess what? When you were born, you were really bendy. The truth is, what most people would consider extreme flexibility—the splits, full lotus, or wheel pose—is merely natural range of motion.

If you doubt this, spend an afternoon with any 10-year-old kid, and you'll be reminded that we were ALL naturally flexible at one time. We've just lost it.

2. YOU DON'T LEARN FLEXIBILITY IN YOGA CLASS

Here's a sad fact: if you think yoga classes are all about stretching flexibility, then you're wrong. Anthony taught me that **most yoga poses _demonstrate_ rather than _develop_ flexibility.** I'd never have guessed this because it's so counterintuitive, but Anthony said *"Yoga is an amazing holistic, spiritual practice; but if you're really stiff and you don't like it, you don't need yoga. You need to stretch!"*

3. FOOD & FLEXIBILITY GO HAND-IN-HAND

"It's possible to eat junk food and improve your flexibility," Anthony said, "but if you really want to increase your stretching flexibility fast, you need to eat less junk and take nutritional supplements every day to make up for what your body is missing."

To think that if you stretch more you'll become more flexible is like saying if you eat less, you'll lose weight. In theory, this is true, but in the real world, it just doesn't work like that. **_To lose weight, you've got to EAT RIGHT and to get flexible you've got to stretch right and eat foods loaded with nutrients!_**

MYTH vs. REALITY

Throw out your anatomy books! When I was really stiff, I spent a couple hundred dollars on *Amazon.com* buying incredibly complex books on yoga anatomy and stretching flexibility. I was trying to figure out what exactly was going on inside me that made my body so inflexible.

OK, I'll admit it. I'm a slow learner.

I read nine books and attended two different anatomy workshops before I realized that learning theory was a waste of time. Flexibility can be summed up in one sentence. Are you ready?

"Flexibility is determined by the length and elasticity of your connective tissues."

Sound too simple? Well, if you'd like, go read a stack of books like I did, but I guarantee that you'll come to the same conclusion. Still not convinced?

Q: Why are my hamstrings so stiff?
A: Your hamstrings are short and tight.

Q: Why is my back so stiff?
A: Your shoulders, upper back muscles, and hip flexors are short and tight.

Q: Why can't I do full lotus?
A: Guess what? The connective tissues surrounding your hips are short and tight.

Q: Is flexibility genetic?
A: *No*

Q: But my mom isn't flexible either!
A: *90% of the general public is stiff... but it's still not genetic.*

Q: My legs are really long; doesn't that make it more difficult to touch my toes?
A: *No.*

Q: My torso is really short; doesn't that make it impossible for me to do backbends?
A: *No.*

Q: I have big thighs; doesn't that mean full lotus pose will be impossible?
A: *Your thighs are not the problem.*

Q: My doctor gave me stretches to do for my back—but they didn't work!
A: *Your doctor doesn't know squat about stretching.*

Q: But my doctor specializes in sports medicine!
A: *Ask him to touch his toes, bend backwards, and do a twist. If he's a bendy guy—fine, listen to him. These people mean well, I'm sure, but 90% of doctors and physical therapists are just as stiff as you.*

Q: I used to be able to do the splits when I was a kid. Why can't I do it anymore?
A: *You used to have loose and limber connective tissues, but now they're tight and short. This is almost always caused by inactivity or repetitive motion activities like swinging a golf club, typing on a computer, or jogging without stretching.*

Q: I saw this stretching machine on TV one night... do you think that it will help?
A: *No. I think it'll hurt. Don't waste any more time.*

Here's the straight story. If your muscles are tight and short, you'll have trouble touching your toes. If they're long and limber, you can learn to put your foot behind your head. The point is, stop worrying about why you're stiff and ***start focusing on getting flexible now!***

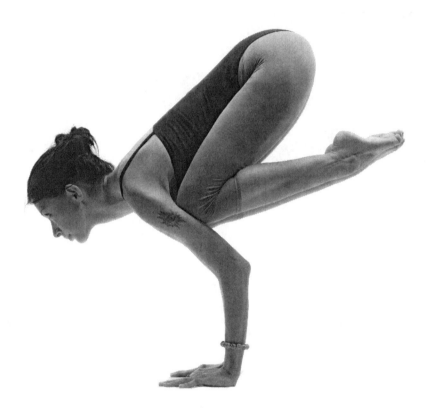

"When the winds of change blow, some people
build walls and others build windmills."
~ *Chinese Proverb*

IMPROVING FLEXIBILITY

We've concluded that there isn't much mystery surrounding the anatomy of flexibility, but when it comes to exactly HOW to increase your stretching flexibility, there are dozens of theories and seemingly conflicting approaches.

Before we get started with stretches, it's important to understand the three primary types of stretching flexibilities.

DYNAMIC FLEXIBILITY

Think of Bruce Lee doing a roundhouse kick! This is an active movement that brings the joints and connective tissues through a full range of motion. Imagine a golfer swinging a 3-iron, a rock climber heaving his leg up onto a high foot hold, or a soccer player doing a flying kick for the ball.

Dynamic flexibility movements are usually done at around *80% of maximum flexibility—and any more than this would be unsafe.*

STATIC FLEXIBILITY

Ever practiced Tai Chi? This "strong-yet-still" flexibility is the type you also see runners practicing when they stretch before a race. Their muscles are engaged (at least to some degree) while they hold a specific pose for a long period of time. Bikram Yoga, for example, is an entire yoga system based on static flexibility stretches with each pose held for 30-60 seconds or longer.

Static flexibility postures are usually practiced at around <u>85% of maximum flexibility</u>, and again, more than this will often lead to injury.

PASSIVE FLEXIBILITY

Ask a dancer to touch her toes, and you'll see passive flexibility in action. This "wet noodle" type of flexibility is also seen in young children or in people who are just "naturally flexible."

Passive flexibility is practiced with little or no muscular energy at all, essentially allowing your body weight and gravity to gently lengthen your muscles and connective tissues. Hence, the "wet noodle" effect.

Passive flexibility poses are usually practiced at around <u>90% of maximum</u> flexibility, and as students progress, it's possible to practice safely at <u>100% maximum flexibility</u> in every single stretch.

SO WHICH ONE IS THE BEST?

All three flexibility types are great, and a balance between the three is ideal. But here, since we're mainly interested in increasing the mobility of certain areas of the body like the back, hips, or shoulders, *passive flexibility exercises tend to be the most effective in rapidly opening the body safely.*

Here's why: you could stretch out your hamstrings by doing multiple sets of round-house kicks, but chances are good that you'd hurt yourself and look pretty stupid in the process!

And the truth is, once you use passive flexibility exercises to overcome your serious blocks, then both static and dynamic flexibility tend to be much easier to learn.

So first we create a flexible, open body, and then we try to kick like Bruce Lee! Does that make sense?

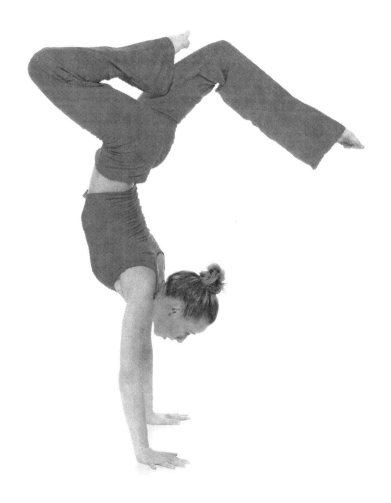

"Yoga helped reduce the number and severity
of injuries I suffered. As preventative medicine,
it's unequaled."
~ *Kareem Abdul-Jabbar*

FOOD & FLEXIBILITY

I KNOW WHAT YOU HAD FOR DINNER LAST NIGHT!

Every yoga teacher knows what you ate for dinner because as soon as you start to sweat, you stink of it! The vodka Redbull, the French onion crisps, the popcorn with artificial butter—all that gunk oozes out between your shoulder blades during sun salutations and collects in a sweat-puddle in your navel while you do bridge pose.

It's in your hair, on your breath, and all over your yoga mat every time you move! Aside from being disgusting, ***junk foods make stretching exercises and yoga poses more difficult.*** Really? Yes, really!

YOU ARE WHAT YOU EAT

Let's look at what happens when you eat an unhealthy meal like Chinese take-out washed down with two cans of beer (one of my old favorites) every night for dinner.

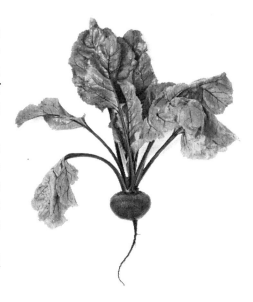

Now, let's suppose you weigh somewhere in the ballpark of 140-160 lbs. In this scenario, take a guess at what 25-35% of your body is made of?

Kung Pao chicken and Budweiser!

25-35% IS A LOT!

Here's what happens: you certainly do burn some of this "food" for energy, transforming whatever nutrients it contains into muscles, connective tissues, and body fat—and then, in an ideal world, you sweat, burp, or urinate out whatever toxic sludge is left.

But if your system is overworked or overloaded, the toxins in that unhealthy dinner—the trans fats, processed sugars, and alcohol—all get dumped into your body fat or muscle tissues!

It doesn't take a genius to realize that if your body is bogged down with crap foods, there's a good chance that it's going to feel and perform like crap too! Think about it.

FRESH & NATURAL

Dharma Mittra, the iconic New York City yoga teacher, once said: *"If you want to feel alive, eat live food."* And he's right!

Fresh, natural foods are the stepping stones on the path of least resistance to a flexible body. Remember, babies are flexible, you <u>were</u> flexible, and you can be flexible again—but you need to make some changes. Cleaning up your diet is a good place to begin.

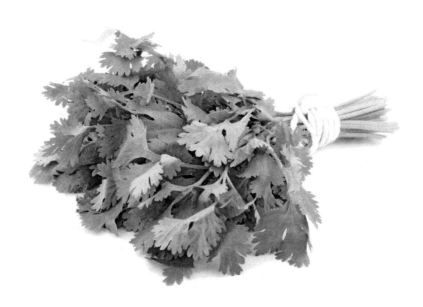

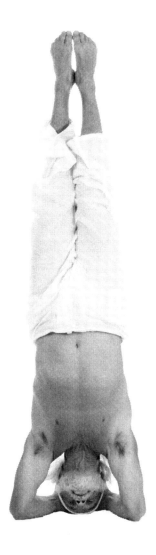

"Yoga practice is the willful effort to restrain the
five activities of the mind and abide in
a state of stillness."
~ *Patanjali*

FLEXIBILITY SUPERFOODS

There are some foods you can eat that will literally make you feel healthier and more limber within 24 hours. Here's the shortlist:

- ✓ **Spirulina** – freshwater blue-green algae
- ✓ **Chlorella** – freshwater blue-green algae
- ✓ **Barley Grass** – juice/extract of sprouted barley grass
- ✓ **Wheatgrass** – juice/extract of sprouted wheatgrass
- ✓ **Green Juices** – juice from any dark, leafy green vegetable
- ✓ **Raw Greens** – kale, chard, spinach
- ✓ **All Seaweeds** (un-salted) – arame, kombu, kelp

WHY GREENS MAKE YOU FLEXIBLE

No one is 100% sure why greens make you flexible, but there are some good theories floating around. First of all, you'll notice all of the foods above are dark green in color. Green is the color of chlorophyll, and chlorophyll is the blood of plants that some believe helps the body absorb oxygen. The theory goes like this:

More Greens = More Oxygen = More Energy, Strength & Flexibility

Dark green vegetables are also loaded with minerals that play an important role in water retention, metabolism, and overall health. Greens contain easily absorbed amino acids (proteins) which may also contribute to their "bendy body" effects on people.

Last but not least, dark green veggies all have **high water content, and water, as you'll learn, is THE most important thing of all.**

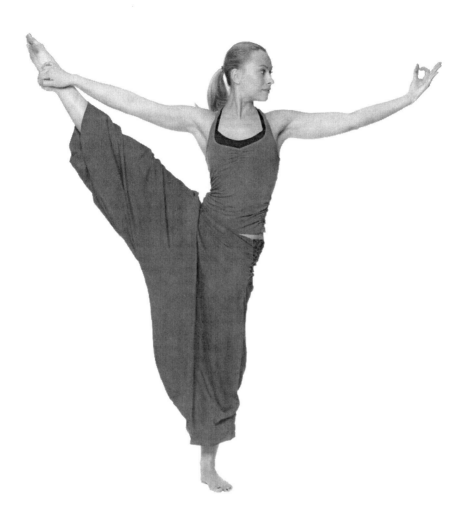

"Yoga is your natural state."
~ *Sharon Gannon*

DRINK MORE WATER

Did you know that 95% of headaches are caused by dehydration? And the same percentage holds true for hangovers and constipation. Sound crazy? It's true! I've run private and group juice fasting programs for years, and it's always amazing how fantastic people feel just 3 hours into the fast.

How can people feel so much better after just 3 hours? Well, by 12 noon, my juice fasters have already drunk 2 liters of liquid (a mixture of juice, water, and nutritional supplements). Simply drinking more water enables most people to feel a huge improvement in their health!

In addition, during a juice fast, _everyone_ feels more flexible within 24 hours because the added liquid provides their bodies with natural lubrication! More liquid in the body also means greater elasticity in the muscles and connective tissues, plus the water provides your system with an effective means of nutrient delivery and waste management.

More Water = More Elasticity in Muscles & Connective Tissues

CAFFEINE MAKES YOU STIFF

Aside from drinking more water for flexibility, you also need to stop drinking so much caffeine, whether it's coffee, tea, or sodas. I used to drink 12 Diet Cokes a day (I'm not joking), so I know first-hand how hard it can be to quit.

To make things worse, most people are totally ignorant of the fact that they're drinking caffeinated beverages all day long. Believe it or not, there is now even a brand of caffeinated beer.

So if you're serious about your flexibility, at the very least, **cut way back on your caffeine intake, and you'll notice the difference immediately.**

Caffeine = Less Water = Sluggish Digestion = Stiffness & Pain

EAT YOUR WATER!

Aside from consuming at least 2 liters of water per day (I often drink 4-6 liters), you also need to *eat your water too!* How do you eat water? You eat foods that have a really high water content... yup, you guessed it! Fruits and vegetables.

Fresh, raw, and organic produce is best, but steamed or lightly sautéed veggies are fine too. The water in fresh produce is even easier for the body to absorb than bottled water because it comes packaged with nature's little helpers: vitamins, minerals, and phyto-nutrients—plus you don't have to think about it!

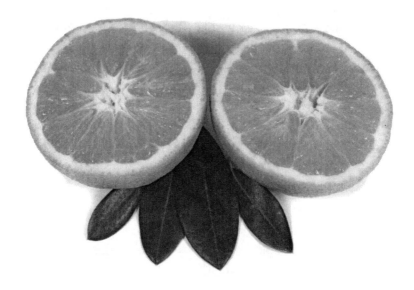

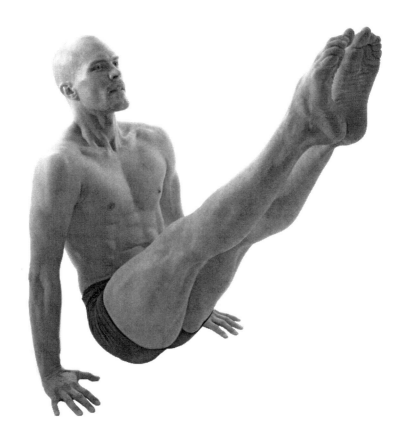

"Do your practice and all is coming."
~ *Sri K. Pattabhi Jois*

THE BAD FOODS

E at the wrong foods, and you'll feel it immediately. Certain foods will slow you down; others will make you stiff and sore within hours. The point of this isn't to make you obsessed over what you eat, but rather to increase your awareness of the consequences that certain foods have on your body.

Here's the shortlist of foods to avoid:

- ✓ **Coffee, Tea, Sodas.** Caffeine is death to stretching. Water is your most important resource, and caffeine acts as a diuretic, draining you of this essential fluid.

- ✓ **Processed Sugar.** Sugar suppresses your immune system, gives you wild mood swings, and can adversely affect your physical ability.

- ✓ **White Bread/White Rice.** These foods form mucous in the body, and mucous makes you stiff and sluggish by literally clogging up your system.

- ✓ **Dairy.** Take one sip of milk and you can feel the phlegm forming in your throat immediately. In India, the cow is sacred and milk is a staple; since yoga came from India, many yoga teachers will lecture you about the benefits of milk and yogurt. Don't listen. I assure you, they've missed the boat!

  That phlegm you feel in the back of your throat is mucous, and dairy is notorious for producing TONS of it all throughout the body. Gooey, glue-like mucous blocks your sinuses, slows digestions, makes you prone to illness—plus it makes you really stiff.

This idea may offend you if milk is one of your comfort foods—something your mother gave you as a child. But let's face it: you're not five years old anymore, and your body doesn't deal with lactose the way it used to.

I'm not trying to start a war, but I am asking you to keep an open mind. Lose the milk, yogurt, and ice cream and watch how deeply you can backbend. Don't take my word for it. Put it to the test.

✓ **Meat.** Meat can take days to digest and the more gunk in your gastrointestinal tract, the more stiff you'll feel. Period.

✓ **Soy & Whey Protein Powders.** Popular health advice tells us we need 100-200 grams of protein per day. Not only is this untrue—it's dangerous. Protein is difficult to digest (strains the liver) and excessive amounts lead to dehydration and acid build-up.

If you do need more protein in your diet (10% of your calories is a good base) because you are traveling or too busy to prepare healthy veggie proteins like broccoli, spinach, raw nuts or seeds, then try Yoga Protein by YOGABODY (sprouted brown rice protein). Learn more here: www.YogaProtein.com

✓ **Deep Fried Anything.** Unhealthy fats act like glue in the body, blocking cellular respiration and throwing the proverbial monkey wrench into your system. Cold-pressed vegetable fats are great (olive oil, coconut oil, sesame oil, etc.), but stay away from cheap, highly processed oils like corn, canola, and soybean.

✓ **Artificial Sweeteners & Additives.** The research on these sweet-tasting, zero-calorie powders is not definitive, but just read the warning labels on any sugar-free products and you'll see why they appear on my *"Foods to Avoid"* list. Neurotoxins, anyone? I think I'll pass. Worse yet, many doctors now believe that the "taste" of sugar substitutes can trigger the same insulin reaction in the body as real sugar.

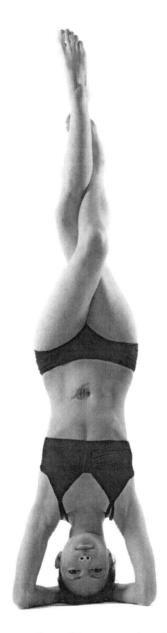

"The energy accumulated in practice has a lot to do with
my ability to get clarity about the reality of things."
~ *John Friend*

THE YOGABODY DIET

I've taught nutrition both privately and to groups since 2002, and I'm always refining and simplifying my dietary recommendations so that it's easier for people to eat healthfully without obsessing, weighing everything, and counting calories.

I've been 100% vegan for a very long time, so obviously, you'll see my suggestions are skewed in that direction. But please know that I've done my research, and more importantly, I've done heavy experimentation, mostly on myself.

Before I switched to a plant-based diet, I tried 7 extremely strict dietary regimes including *The Zone, Atkins, a Ketogenic Diet, and a 100% Raw Food Diet.* When I say I "tried" these diets, I really mean it.

I strictly followed *The Zone* for 2.5 years (weighing foods, counting calories, etc.), was a strict raw foodist for nearly 2 years, and I ate a purely fat diet (*Ketogenic Diet*) for nearly 2.5 months.

I'm serious about nutrition, and I don't mess around. I'll admit, my views are biased, but not from some theoretical high horse. **My opinions are all based on my own research and years of real-life experiments.** As with everything, I encourage you to draw your own conclusions.

EAT MORE PLANTS

Let's imagine for a moment a chimpanzee, who, genetically speaking, is less than 5% different from humans. This chimp in the jungle doesn't eat at Taco Bell. He doesn't snack on Power Bars or drink protein shakes. Once in awhile, he might swallow larvae or feast on an ant hill, but mostly—like almost all of the time—chimpanzees eat plants.

I'm not calling you a monkey, but let's use basic logic. ***Nature's plant life provides such a wealth of nutrition for strength, energy, and radiant health,*** and yet most of us opt-out, choosing instead the bizarre processed concoctions on supermarket shelves.

The YOGABODY Diet is a return to nature, and I've discovered that of all the foods available to us, those of plant-based origin make most people look and feel their best, again and again, over long periods of time.

DRINK BEER, EAT STEAK & LIVE to be 100?

We all know at least one person who eats terribly, drinks like a fish, and yet somehow enjoys exceptional health. If you're one of these people, God bless you!

If not, I'd really suggest you take a careful look at your diet. Small changes go a long way, and just like money in a savings account, your health compounds itself over time and can make a HUGE difference long term.

EAT YOUR FRUITS & VEGETABLES

At my restaurant in Thailand, I was amazed at how many adults don't like vegetables. It's difficult for me to believe, but customers would sometimes request that my cooks remove *"anything green"* from their plate. So weird!

When you were little, your mom probably told you to eat your fruits and vegetables, and surprise, surprise—she was right. Fruits and vegetables are kick-ass foods for a number of reasons, but here's a shortlist.

Fruits & Vegetables Contain:

- ✓ 40-90% water
- ✓ easy-to-digest protein
- ✓ healthy fats
- ✓ complex carbohydrates (the good kind)
- ✓ fiber
- ✓ vitamins
- ✓ minerals

✓ phyto-nutrients
✓ active enzymes

Plus, fruits and vegetables are nearly impossible to overeat; they give you long-lasting energy, promote digestive health, and are some of the most beautiful and delicious foods on the planet.

EVEN MEAT COMES FROM THE EARTH

The truth is, all edible foods originated in the soil—even beef! Think about it... the cow eats grass, which it converts into muscle that the butcher cuts off his rump for our barbequing pleasure.

In theory, this system sounds pretty slick: the cow does all the grunt work out in the field, and all we have to do is bop him over the head and fire up the grill.

Unfortunately, the law of bio-magnification complicates things because all the toxins in the environment get concentrated in the animals that are highest on the food chain.

Admittedly, a cow is not THAT high on the food chain—but compared to a piece of broccoli, the cow is a god. ***Here's how it works:*** the cow drinks from polluted water, chomps on pesticide-laden grain, and gets pumped full of antibiotics for its entire (short-lived) life—and then passes all these goodies on to us every time we eat a hamburger or a T-bone steak.

For this reason—and an entire book's worth of other reasons—I always recommend people reduce the amount of meat in their diet to 10% or less of their total calories.

The exact same is true of dairy products, and if you're going to pick one or the other, eliminate dairy from your diet first because you'll notice the health benefits straight away. Plus, it's believed that dairy cows suffer more than beef cattle, so you'll earn yourself some happy cow karma points too.

EAT AT THE BOTTOM OF THE FOOD CHAIN

As a general rule, the closer to the bottom of the food chain you eat, the better. This obviously includes fruits, vegetables, nuts, and seeds—but don't forget seaweeds, mushrooms, and sprouts!

Biologically, our bodies understand how to process and eliminate most plant foods. *Fruits and vegetables, for example, are difficult to overeat because our bodies naturally let us know when we've had enough.* Plant foods promote healthy bowel movements and are also loaded with very easy to absorb vitamins, minerals, proteins, fats, and carbohydrates.

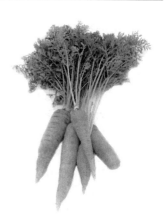

KEEP NATURAL FOODS NATURAL

If you take plant foods out of their natural state, our bodies often don't know how to react. Imagine for a moment, a big bowl of raw broccoli. This is a nice snack, but I assure you, it will leave you feeling quite full. Take that same broccoli, batter and deep fry it—and suddenly your body has no idea what to do. The smell of fat triggers a primal craving, and you go crazy and eat the whole bowl and still want more.

For this reason, try to minimize the amount of processed foods you eat. *The easiest way to do this is to make sure that <u>most</u> of the foods you eat actually resemble something that grows from the ground.*

SO WHAT DO I EAT?

Simplicity is essential when it comes to eating, and the pie chart below is one of the easiest tools for figuring out what to eat to maintain health and balance. To use this graph, imagine that each plate of food you eat is split into three pieces:

- 70% of your plate should contain water-based foods
- 20% should be concentrated foods
- 10% can be dry foods

What Should I Eat?

Dry Foods
10%

Water-Based Foods
70%

Concentrated Foods
20%

Keep in mind, eating a meal or snack of *only* water-based foods is totally healthy too!

EAT 70% WATER-BASED FOODS

The planet is about 70% water, your body is about 70% water, and likewise, the healthiest foods tend to have a similar water content.

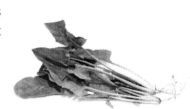

- Fruits
- Vegetables
- Sprouts
- Beans
- Sea Vegetables (kombu, arame, nori, etc.)

EAT 20% CONCENTRATED FOODS

Concentrated foods are excellent for you, but contain less water and are more potent (in terms of calories) than water-based foods. For this reason, we want to be sure to eat these foods every day but in smaller quantities.

- Cold-pressed oils
- Raw nuts & seeds
- Olives
- Nut butters (tahini, almond butter, etc.)
- Tempeh and tofu
- Dry fruit (raisins, apricots, dates, figs, etc.)
- Whole grains & cereals
- Oatmeal

EAT 10% DRY FOODS

Dry foods aren't *bad* for you; they're just not that great for you. Sometimes referred to as *"empty calories,"* dry foods contain densely-packed carbohydrates that need to be taken in moderation. ***Excessive dry foods can cause weight gain, food cravings, and sluggish digestion.***

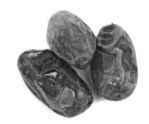

Again, these are <u>not bad</u> foods; you just need to eat them in smaller quantities.

- Rice
- Noodles
- Wheat (bread, muffins, rolls, etc.)

BUT I LOVE RED WINE AND CHOCOLATE CAKE!

I'm not asking you to give up your favorite foods or eat like a monk. Be creative and think outside the box when it comes to your nutrition! Try some of the changes I've suggested, and then decide what works for you.

I've seen chronic allergies disappear in days when students gave up milk; I've seen blood pressure drop overnight when all animal fats were eliminated from students' diets; and I've seen pizza-faced skin go completely clear in 1 week simply by eating 70% water-based foods and taking the nutritional supplement MSM.

And get this: I've also received hundreds of emails from stretching students who say they feel more flexible within 24-hours on the YOGABODY Diet. So think about it. Conduct your own experiments, make some changes, and see what happens.

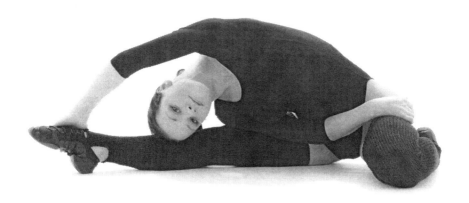

"The beauty is that people often come here for the
stretch, and leave with a lot more."
~ *Liza Ciano*

NUTRITIONAL SUPPLEMENTS

I used to believe that I should be able to get all the nutrients I needed from the foods I ate. After all, I was eating extremely healthfully. I'd given up coffee, sugar, wheat, meat, and dairy. My entire diet consisted of fresh, organic produce, juice, and home-grown sprouts—and yet, I wasn't getting everything I needed.

How do I know this? Well, I snipped off some of my hair and sent it to a lab to be analyzed for minerals and toxins. It turned out that I was deficient in 5 important trace minerals, including zinc and selenium.

Needless to say, I was surprised, and it instantly confirmed everything that Anthony had taught me. Despite the fact that I was eating an amazing diet, I didn't have all the building blocks my body needed to grow and change the way I wanted it to.

So what did I do?

I started taking Anthony's recommended supplement mix, and later, I found all-natural alternatives for all the same nutrients. Then, I created the YOGABODY Stretch formula to make my life easier (basically, I stuck six nutritional supplements all in one pill).

Here's what it contains:
- **MSM** (methylsulfonylmethane)
- **Triple Green Blend** (organic spirulina, organic chlorella & barley grass juice extract)
- **Ultra-Sorb Vitamin C** (ascorbic acid buffered with calcium ascorbate)
- **Trace Mineral Uptake Enhancers**

MSM (Methylsulfonylmethane)

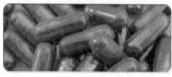

MSM originates in the ocean, but is extracted from the lignin of pine trees. The MSM I use is 99.9% pure, making it indistinguishable from the MSM found in broccoli, peppers, Brussels sprouts, onions, asparagus, cabbage, and mother's milk.

MSM acts as a ***powerful antioxidant and healing source*** of natural sulfur.

Why sulfur? Stretching puts a great deal of stress on your muscles, joints, tendons, and ligaments; and sulfur, which is found in every cell of our bodies, is an essential building block for promoting elasticity, strength, and the general health of our connective tissues.

For stretching students, MSM has been shown to ***relieve inflammation and reduce recovery time.***

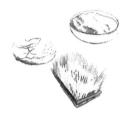

TRIPLE GREEN BLEND (Certified Organic Spirulina, Certified Organic Chlorella, Pesticide/ Herbicide/Fungicide-free Barley Grass Juice Extract)

Spirulina (fresh water algae) delivers a whopping dose of B vitamins, Iron, and the essential fat GLA.

Chlorella (fresh water algae) is packed with chlorophyll, also known as *"the blood of plants,"* and is believed to have powerful blood/body cleansing properties.

Chlorella is also known to ***boost energy*** and aid in the natural elimination of heavy metals and other toxins from the body.

Barley Grass Juice Extract, the ultimate green food, is excellent for stretching students because of its high levels of beta-carotene, calcium, and iron.

UTLRA-SORB VITAMIN C
(Ascorbic Acid with Calcium Ascorbate)
Vitamin C is well-known for its ability to
boost the immune system, fight free radicals,
and ward off illness, but researchers are
now discovering that Vitamin C also plays
a key role in regeneration of tissues.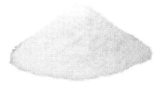

Vitamin C is naturally acidic, so I've buffered it with alkalizing calcium ascorbate which makes it easier to digest and absorb.

Recent medical studies suggest that MSM and Vitamin C work synergistically to boost the immune system, fight aging, and reduce recovery time.

TRACE MINERAL UPTAKE ENHANCERS
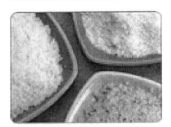 Trace minerals like cobalt, selenium, magnesium, and zinc play a vital role in dozens of metabolic processes such as tissue growth, healthy metabolism, and proper water retention.

These minerals work in collaboration with other vitamins and phyto-nutrients, increasing their absorption and boosting their effectiveness.

In the past, the earth was naturally rich in minerals, but over-cultivation has led to mineral deficiencies in the soil that carry over into our bodies. To ensure nutrient balance, trace minerals are essential, and a daily dose of YOGABODY Stretch does the trick.

WHERE DO YOU GET YOUR PROTEIN?

When you start eating a mostly plant-based diet, people will constantly ask you, "Where do you get your protein?" Entire books have been written on protein in vegetarian diets, so I won't attempt to include the full body of research here.

But as a former protein junkie and skeptical vegetarian, I've researched this issue extensively. I've personally interviewed two different medical doctors (one holistic, one conventional), met with over two dozen long-time vegetarians, and read every piece of research on the subject I could find because it seems like a valid concern.

The high-protein mass hysteria that dominates pop health today originated with a weight loss book called, *Dr. Atkins' Diet Revolution* in the early 1970's. Dr. Atkins' weight loss protocol involves consuming copious amounts of high-protein foods (30%+ of total calories) and avoiding carbohydrates.

Here's the problem: Weight loss and health are not always the same thing. For example, if you take laxatives and smoke a pack of cigarettes each day, you'll probably lose weight—but that's obviously not healthy.

It's now believed that diets which are unnaturally high in protein (30%+ of total calories) tax the liver, put the body in a constant acidic state, leach vital minerals from your system, and can lead to degenerative illnesses. Dr. Atkins himself was 255 lbs., clinically obese, and suffered from heart disease and hypertension before he passed away in 2003.

Modern versions of the "Atkin's Diet" have appeared over the years, most notably Dr. Barry Sear's book, *The Zone*. And while "The Zone Diet," recommends healthier sources for protein (like lean meats and soy products), the recommended intake of protein at 30%+ remains highly controversial.

New research suggests that most people need just 10% of dietary calories to come from protein. As reported in his book, *The China Study*, T. Colin Campbell, Ph.D., discovered that the healthiest people in the world consume a low protein, mostly plant-based diet. Campbell came to this conclusion after exhaustive research that included a "survey of death rates for twelve different kinds of cancer for more than 2,400 counties and 880 million of their citizens" conducted jointly by Cornell University, Oxford University, and the Chinese Academy of Preventive Medicine over the course of twenty years.

Based on his findings, Campbell deduced that a diet of approximately 10% protein is optimal for most people for long-term health and wellness.

Plant foods, eaten in variety, contain complete proteins just like meat. There are 22 standard amino acids (protein building blocks) in foods, 9 of which are essential (must be eaten, body cannot create). The remaining amino acids are non-essential, meaning they can be synthesized from other macro nutrients.

All 22 standard amino acids are abundant and widely available in many plant food combinations with extremely high quantities found in foods such as quinoa, buckwheat, hempseed, amaranth, dark green vegetables, legumes, nuts, and seeds.

Despite the abundance of protein in a plant-based diet, some vegetarians and busy people still fail to meet their minimal protein requirements (even at just 10% of total calories) because they are in a rush and end up eating carbohydrate-based meals like sandwiches, pastas, fruit, biscuits, snack foods, and rice dishes.

SHOULD YOU TAKE A PROTEIN SUPPLEMENT?

On a home cooked, low-protein, plant-based diet, it's fairly easy to get adequate amounts of amino acids (protein building blocks). So if you prepare most of your meals yourself and are a big vegetable eater; chances are, you don't need to worry about supplementing.

The challenge arises when you're too busy to prepare your meals. My experience is that almost everyone falls into this category at least a few times each month—and many of us every day.

Consider taking 15-30 grams of supplemental protein if:
- You eat outside your own home at least 1x per day
- You travel often
- Your tendency is to "carb out" on bread, pasta, or rice
- You know you don't eat enough greens and seeds
- You are physically active or working to overcome a physical injury
- You tend to have very little lean muscle mass
- You are experimenting with a vegetarian, vegan or raw vegan diet for the first time.

Perhaps you have work or family obligations; or maybe you travel often and end up eating out. If this is the case, your diet inevitably becomes dominated by simple carbohydrates. This is when I find it extremely helpful to supplement your diet with a plant-based protein supplement—ideally rice protein as it's hypoallergenic, easy to digest, and the most natural choice.

Let's be clear though: I'm not talking about massive 100 gram protein shakes that body builders chug down after pumping iron. This is a simple 15-30 grams of protein per day added to reach the desired 50-80 grams of protein that is needed for most people to maintain a lean, strong body.

WHAT ABOUT SOY AND WHEY PROTEIN?

Soy protein is often extracted using hexane, an explosive chemical solvent that leaves residues behind—often at dangerously high levels—in soy protein powders and soy products. While whole bean, organic, non-genetically modified soy beans are a great food to include in your diet; the supplements made from soy should be avoided completely.

Soy protein also creates digestive and allergic reactions in a large percentage of users.

Whey protein comes from cow's milk which is almost always tainted with the telltale signs of factory farming. Dairy products commonly contain antibiotics, pesticides, herbicides, hormones, and dioxin.

On the consumer side, whey protein is notorious for causing extremely potent flatulence.

WHAT'S SO GREAT ABOUT RICE PROTEIN?

Brown rice is a naturally-occurring, nutrient-dense grain that is agreeable to nearly every digestive system in the world. As a concentrated protein powder, it's hypoallergenic (no allergies), nearly tasteless, and easy to digest with no gas or digestive issues associated with other protein products. Rice protein delivers maximum absorption, making it the supplement of choice for plant-based amino acids.

WANT TO LEARN MORE?

To learn more about the protein supplement I personally use and recommend please go to: www.YogaProtein.com

WHAT ABOUT VITAMIN B12?

Vitamin B12 is one of the only known nutrients found in animal foods that is almost impossible to find in the plant kingdom, making the question of B12 one of the most controversial and highly-discussed topics among vegetarians worldwide.

To complicate the discussion, B12 deficiency (though not common) occurs almost as often in meat eaters as in vegetarians, probably due to our high-stress lifestyles more than anything else. A B12-rich diet or B12 food supplements are recommended to both vegetarians and non-vegetarians to alleviate the following conditions:

- Lack of energy
- Depression
- Lack of focus
- Asthma
- Sleep disorders
- HIV/AIDS
- Infertility (in men)
- Tinnitus

WHAT IS VITAMIN B12, ANYWAY?

Vitamin B12 is an essential, water-soluble vitamin that is found in a variety of animal foods such as fish, shellfish, meat, and dairy products. In nature, and in nutritional supplements, Vitamin B12 is often combined with other B vitamins in a vitamin B complex to increase absorption and bioavailability. It's unclear whether vegetarian food sources of B12 such as nutritional yeast or fermented foods provide enough bio-available B12 long term, so for those on a plant-based diet, it's smart to supplement with B12 at least occasionally. High-quality B12 supplements are made from a controlled fermentation process and do not contain animal products.

Aside from preventing deficiency, B12 also helps maintain healthy nerve and red blood cells and is needed to make DNA. The human body stores several years' worth of vitamin B12, so while chronic deficiency is not common, it does happen. And since supplementing with B12 (at least occasionally) can have such positive benefits, many yoga students find it's a great addition to any conscious, healthy diet.

BENEFITS OF B12 (from diet or supplementation)

If you're transitioning to a plant-based diet, the responsible thing to do is ensure you're either eating some B12-rich animal foods (such as eggs or chicken) or else take a simple, B vitamin complex supplement. Reported benefits include:
- Increased attention, clarity and focus
- Increased energy and stamina
- Natural mood elevation

WANT TO LEARN MORE?

Many B vitamin supplements contain yeast and can give you terrible gas and bloating. To learn more about the yeast-free, liquid form of bio-available B12 that I use, called Liquid Clarity-B, please visit: www.YogaB12.com

DO I NEED to EAT FISH?

F ish are often considered the healthiest of animal foods because they are low in saturated fat, high in protein, and rich in Omega-3 essential fatty acids (EFA's). Unfortunately, there are many problems with commercial fish that are only getting worse. But before we dive deeper into the question of whether or not to eat fish, let's take a closer look at why Omega-3 fatty acids are getting so much attention and what the real story is about essential fats, fish, and your health.

WHAT ARE ESSENTIAL FATTY ACIDS (EFA'S)?

Your body needs all 3 macro nutrients—carbohydrates, protein, and fat—to be healthy, and even if you are not eating a well-balanced diet, your body will do its best to correct that. For example, if you eat nothing but fruit—even for weeks at a time—your body can easily change that fructose (fruit sugar) into fat, but it cannot create essential fats like Omega-3. So that's why it's essential that you eat these lipids regularly.

The two most common essential fats are Omega-3 and Omega-6. Omega-6 is readily available (and often over-consumed) because almost all vegetable oils are loaded with it, while Omega-3 is relatively rare in both the plant and animal kingdoms.

WHY IS OMEGA-3 SO GOOD?

The laundry list of Omega-3 fatty acids' benefits is so widely recognized that food and dietary supplementation is now recommended by both mainstream and alternative health professionals all over the world.

Here's a short list of the reported benefits, many of which have undergone the scrutiny of the US Food and Drug Administration:
- Reduces triglyceride levels
- Helps reverse heart disease
- Promotes healthy bowels
- Supports neurological health
- Contributes to emotional health (mood)
- Boosts immune function
- Balances blood sugar
- Fights off cancer

SO WHAT ABOUT FISH?

Assuming you're eating a well-balanced diet with healthy quantities of essential fatty acids from plant sources such as chia seeds (salvia hispanica), flaxseeds, or walnuts, then you certainly don't need to rely on fish for your Omega-3 needs.

If you are not vegetarian, the richest Omega-3 fish are salmon, herring, mackerel, anchovies, and sardines. Of these five, only salmon is commonly available fresh or frozen. The others are most-often canned, processed, salty foods that should be avoided.

If you live in a region where there is fresh or frozen wild-caught salmon available, this might be a good option for you. The biggest (and growing) concerns in regards to fish for non-vegetarians and vegetarians alike are (1) the environmental impact of overfishing which is affecting 70-80% of the planet (seriously, fish are going extinct), (2) the increasing levels of mercury and other toxins found in fish due to pollution (fish are like sponges for water pollutants), and (3) the high cost of eating wild-caught fish on a regular basis (fresh salmon daily is not cheap).

WHAT ARE THE OTHER OPTIONS?

You can now find poultry enhanced with natural Omega-3 fatty acids from farmers who feed flaxseeds to their chickens to increase their EFA levels. The poultry industry and poultry products are not on anyone's shortlist for health, but if you're going to eat them, these naturally-enhanced animal foods are a healthier choice and often come from organic and free range farms.

Alternatively, you can just eat salvia hispanica or flaxseeds and skip the animal farming industry altogether which is my personal preference and recommendation.

WANT TO LEARN MORE?

To learn more about salvia hispanica seeds, the veggie source that I use for Omega-3 (a.k.a. "Yoga Seeds"), please visit: www.YogaOmega3.com

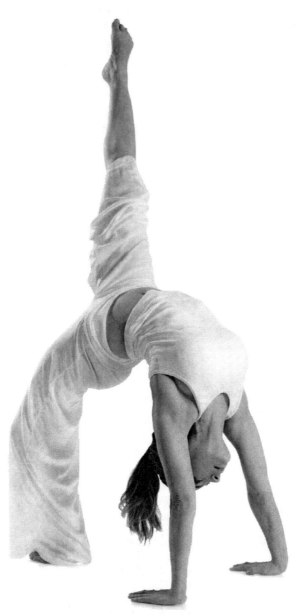

"I did not come to yoga to stretch. I came to live."
~ *Maya Breuer*

HOW TO STRETCH

If you go to a sports medicine doctor or physical therapist for flexibility, he'll most likely recommend Proprioceptive Neuromuscular Facilitation (PNF) which involves a strength-to-stretch exercise routine where short bursts of muscular contraction are followed by brief periods of deep stretching.

Go to an Ashtanga Yoga class, and your teacher will tell you to hold each yoga pose for around 5 breaths; while in Iyengar Yoga classes, you'll often hold poses for 5 minutes!

And if you Google search for *"flexibility systems"*, you'll find all sorts of medieval stretching (torture?) machines and oversized rubber bands that are just plain scary!

SO WHAT'S THE BEST WAY TO INCREASE YOUR FLEXIBILITY?

Here's the sad truth. Most people *never* stretch, so *anything* you do will be helpful, and almost any safe method of stretching can be effective... eventually.

But since you're reading this, my guess is that "eventually" to you is probably synonymous with "never".

So I'm going to assume that you'd like to speed up the process with an optimized stretching routine that will help you obtain the maximum mobility in the shortest possible time. Sound good?

You're in luck! The stretching exercises I'm going to teach you are unconventional and a bit awkward, but they'll most certainly help you get flexible safely and quickly using highly-targeted passive stretches! To put it simply, this is an easy system for safely opening your body fast.

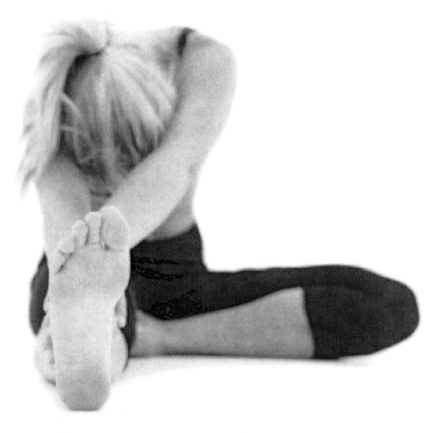

"You can enter yoga, or the path of yoga, only when you are totally frustrated with your own mind as it is. If you are still hoping that you can gain something through your mind, yoga is not for you."

~ *Osho*

GRAVITY POSES

My yoga friend, Anthony, taught me that true flexibility is learned at home and that the best way to improve is to use these really weird yoga postures that he called Gravity Poses. They're really simple to do, but be sure to do them <u>exactly</u> as instructed.

SO WHAT ARE GRAVITY POSES?

Take a look at the palm tree in the picture below. You can see that the constant force of the wind blows the tree to the right, while the steady force of gravity pushes it toward the ground.

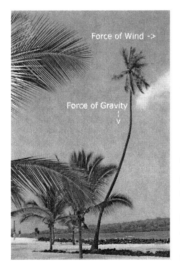

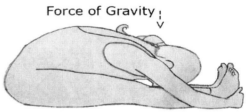

So what does this have to do with stretching? Gravity is <u>strong enough</u> to bend wood significantly, but <u>gentle enough</u> not to break it. ***This balance is essential for maximizing your stretching flexibility safely!***

HOW TO PRACTICE GRAVITY POSES

Forget what you've learned in yoga and stretching classes, and follow these three instructions carefully.

1. **RELAX.** Use as little energy as possible in whatever stretching exercise you're doing. Don't move, wiggle, bounce, or pull. Relax completely!

2. **DON'T FIGHT GRAVITY.** Let nature's gentle force press you down.

3. **NOSE-TO-MOUTH BREATHING.** Inhale deeply through your nose and exhale out your mouth. Take in as much air as you can without straining on the inhale, and empty your lungs completely before taking a new breath.

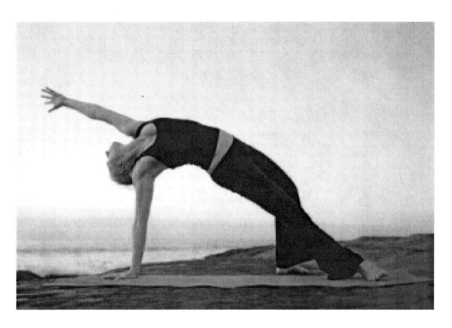

"Anyone who practices can obtain success in
yoga but not one who is lazy. Constant practice
alone is the secret of success."
~ *Swami Svatmarama*

STRETCHING TIPS

WARM UP

The warmer you are before you stretch, the more effective each session will be. Because of the nature of these Gravity Poses, it's completely safe to practice <u>without warming up</u>; but, if at all possible, take a couple minutes to get your heart pumping. It'll make all your stretches more effective.

There are dozens of ways to warm up, but here are four of the easiest that you can do at home in just five short minutes (choose one):

- **Sun Salutations.** 10 yinyasa yoga sun salutations are great for warming up the body.

- **Jumping Jacks.** Do 4 sets of 50 and you'll be good to go!

- **Push Ups.** Pump out 5 sets of 10-20 (depending on your strength) and you'll be very warm.

- **Stair Climb.** Run up and down stairs for about 5 minutes without stopping.

BREATHING

If you've done yoga or pilates before, you've probably been given very clear instructions on breathing. For Gravity Poses, forget what you've learned. Breathe in through <u>your nose</u> deeply, and exhale out through <u>your mouth</u>.

This technique helps to relax and release all the tension in your body, deep down into the connective tissues.

FOLLOW INSTRUCTIONS

I've taught over 1,000 yoga asana classes, so I know how eager people can be to improve their stretching flexibility. However, ***to avoid injury and maximize your benefits,*** you need to <u>follow instructions</u>, be patient, breathe deeply, and relax!

You can't force flexibility. You must finesse it.

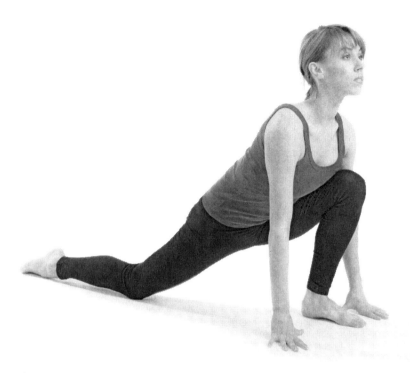

"The same posture, the same sequence, the same meditation... will have entirely different outcomes."
~ *Donna Farhi*

STRETCHING SCHEDULE

WHEN TO STRETCH

You can stretch whenever you like, but first thing in the morning or right before bed are the preferred times. In the mornings, you'll feel more stiff, but you'll progress just as quickly as any other time of the day.

YOGA MAT?

Some people like to use a yoga mat, but it's not neccesarry. You can also use a rug or towel, or even just stretch on the floor. For some postures, you might want to use something to pad your knees.

SCHEDULE

In order to get results, consistency is essential. Stick to <u>at least</u> 15 minutes per day, five days per week. I usually recommend people follow the workweek schedule and take the weekends off, but the truth is, you can stretch every day if you like!

STRETCHING SCHEDULE (suggested)

MONDAY – Target Area: Hamstrings (2 yoga poses)
TUESDAY – Target Area: Hips (2 yoga poses)
WEDNESDAY – Target Area: Shoulders (3 yoga poses)
THURSDAY – Target Area: Back (3 yoga poses)
FRIDAY – Target Area: Wrists, Twists, Ankles (3 yoga poses)

EXTRA STRETCHING

It's important that you do all the poses in each target area before moving on to another area, but it's prefectly acceptable to do 30 minutes of stretching each day by combining days (example: combine days 1&2, then 3&4, etc.).

What you want to avoid is picking and choosing poses from different days and mixing them together, because *each area needs a solid 15 minutes or more of attention before moving on to the next area.*

Day 1 – Hamstrings

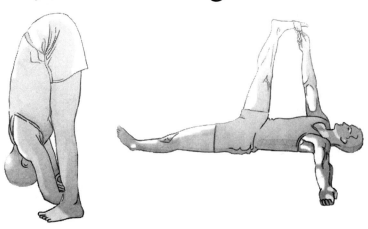

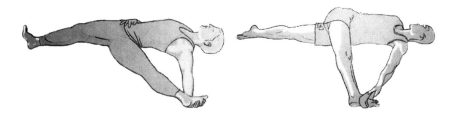

Day 2 – Hips

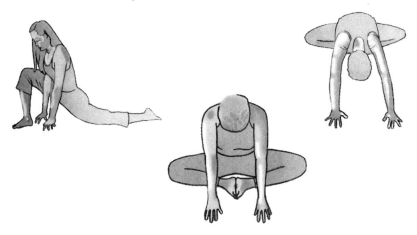

Day 3 – Shoulders

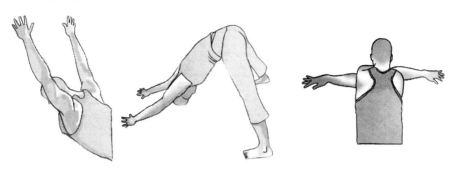

Day 4 – Back

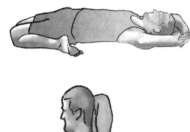

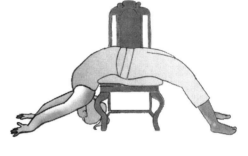

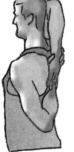

Day 5 – Wrists, Twists, Ankles

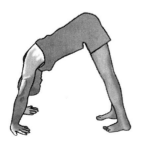
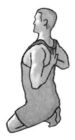
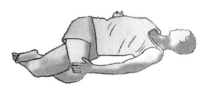

Day 1: Hamstrings

OVERVIEW

The hamstrings refer to a group of muscles located at the back of the thigh. This long group of tissues works in opposition to the quadriceps on the front of the leg.

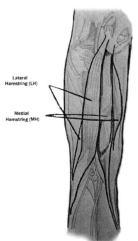

Lateral
Hamstring (LH)

Medial
Hamstring (MH)

When you bend your leg, the hamstring muscles contract and the quadriceps muscles relax. Conversely, when you straighten your leg, the quadriceps muscles contract and the hamstring muscles relax.

SIGNS OF TIGHT HAMSTRINGS

- ✓ Difficulty forward bending
- ✓ Pain in the backs of legs during exercise
- ✓ Pain in lower back during forward bending
- ✓ Bad posture

FIND YOURS NOW!

From standing, bend forward at the hips until you feel a tug at the back of your leg. Using your fingers, you'll easily identify some or all of the hamstring muscles.

WHY THIS IS IMPORTANT

For flexibility, hamstrings are usually the starting point. Tight hamstrings cause all sorts of problems ranging from lower back pain to poor posture. ***When your hamstrings are loose and lean, you'll have better posture, improved physical performance, and reduced risk of injury to your lower back.***

DAY 1: Rag Doll

THE SETUP

1 –   Feet hips-width apart
2 –   Knees <u>slightly</u> bent
3 –   Grab your elbows
4 –   <u>Relax</u> your head completely
5 –   Use as little energy as possible
6 –   Hold for 2-5 minutes

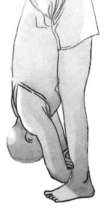

We've all done this posture a million times, but most people never practice it properly, in a way that actually increases stretching flexibility.

Remember this: the hamstrings include 3 massive muscles plus dozens of other connective tissues. Bobbing up and down like joggers in the park isn't going to do squat for your flexibility.

You've got to relax, breathe deeply, <u>bend your knees</u> a little and stay here for as long as you can.

TIPS:
 • Be sure to relax your head & neck.
 • Keep your feet parallel to each other.
 • Don't wiggle or bounce at all.
 • Back off if you feel sharp pain in the lower back.

This is a super simple pose, and when practiced properly it will absolutely amaze you; it's that powerful! Eventually, you want to work up to a 5 minute hold, but don't be a cowboy. Set a goal of 2 minutes and slowly increase over time.

DAY 1: Flamenco

THE SETUP

1 – Lie on your back.

2 – Lift your right leg up and take hold of the foot, either with your right hand, a towel, or belt, holding on with your <u>right hand only</u>.

Note: the leg should be straight so use a towel or belt if needed.

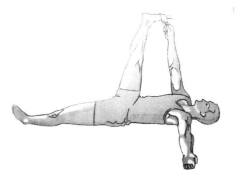

3 – <u>Relax</u> your entire body.

4 – Hold for 3-5 minutes.

5 – Next, using your right hand only, open the leg to the right and hold for 3-5 minutes.

Note: the foot can be off the floor.

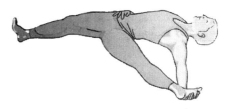

6 – Bring the leg up and cross it over the body, and using the <u>left hand</u>, hold for 3-5 minutes.

Note: the foot can be off the floor.

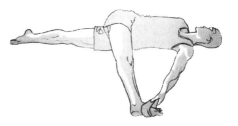

7 – Repeat steps 1-6 on the other side.

 TIPS:
- Both legs should be straight <u>and</u> relaxed at all times.
- Use a towel or belt if needed.
- Do not pull hard on the foot; just allow the natural pull that occurs to help you stretch.
- Do <u>not</u> rest between sides.
- Hold the foot, towel, or belt with <u>one hand only</u>.

This pose can feel very awkward at first, and many people have a tendency to pull on the foot—but don't do it! Lie back, relax, and allow gravity to do the work.

This pose will increase the range of motion in your hamstrings quickly and gently. Eventually, you can spend 30 minutes just moving through variations of this one pose.

Day 2: Hips

The hips are some of the largest joints in the body. So, not surprisingly, they have a huge group of muscles and connective tissues that support them.

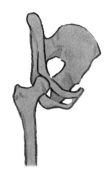

How many different muscles control the hips?

There are different opinions on this, but it's fair to say that there are at least 17 individual muscles including the gluteus, abductors, iliopsoas, and piriformis.

So what does that mean?

Well, when people say, *"I have tight hips,"* often they visualize their actual hip joint (see picture above) as being locked up. This is possible, but not likely. Most people have healthy hip joints, while the muscles in their pelvis, butt, and legs that support the joint are tightened and shortened.

SIGNS OF TIGHT HIPS

- ✓ If sitting cross-legged, your knees are way off the floor.
- ✓ If you cannot squat down deeply without the heels of your feet coming up off the ground.

WHY THIS IS IMPORTANT

When your hips are open, simple activities like tying your shoes, picking something up off the ground, or sitting cross-legged on the floor, become much more comfortable. People with open hips are also better at sports and better dancers.

IMPORTANT NOTE

The more muscles being stretched at once, the more time you'll need to spend in the pose. For this reason, the hip joint is often very stubborn when it comes to increasing your stretching flexibility. ***The trick is consistent, long holds and deep breathing.***

Day 2: The Blaster

THE SETUP

1 – From a push-up position, step your right foot outside your hands and let your left leg rest on the floor behind you.

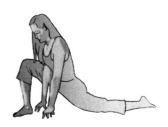

2 – Use your right hand to push the foot forward so that the <u>ankle</u> is either <u>directly below</u> or else <u>in front</u> of the knee.

3 – Turn your right foot slightly angled to the right.

4 – Rest your finger tips or the palms of your hands on the floor in line with your heel (not in front of the heel).

5 – If you feel comfortable, a more advanced option is to drop down so that your elbows, instead of your hands, are on the floor in one line with your heel.

6 – Drop your head and use as little energy as possible.

7 – Hold for 4-5 minutes.

8 – Repeat on the other side.

TIPS:
- Allow gravity to gently move you toward the floor.
- Relax your legs and soften your hip area.
- Let your head drop, heavy like a bowling ball.
- Don't move your feet or your hands.
- You'll need to use your arms or forearms for support, but try to use them as little as possible.

This pose opens the hips like no other. After five minutes here, you won't believe how much mobility you've gained—and it just keeps getting better! ***Remember that your foot must be underneath or further forward than your knee for this to work safely.***

Note: The 17+ muscles supporting your hip are going to need some serious encouragement to loosen up. Wiggling around and changing your position every 10 seconds will only lessen the effectiveness of this powerful posture... so don't move!

Day 2: Butterfly

THE SETUP

1 – Bring the soles of your feet together in front of you.

2 – Scoot your bum forward so it's close to your feet.

3 – Walk your fingers forward on the floor until you reach your maximum.

4 – Relax your arms, head, and entire body completely.

5 – Do not bounce or wiggle.

6 – Be careful with your knees, and if you feel sharp pain, back off.

7 – When you feel resistance, stop moving forward.

8 – Hold for 3-5 minutes.

 TIPS:

- Consciously tell yourself to relax your legs, head, and neck so you're completely soft.
- As you feel your hips relaxing, gently slide your hands forward and then relax again.
- Your head is heavy, so let it hang loose and free.
- If you have trouble leaning forward, place a pillow underneath your bum.

The Butterfly pose can be really awkward, especially if your knees are high off the floor and you can barely fold forward—but don't despair!

After five minutes in this pose, you'll already notice the difference. There's a tendency to bounce with the knees and pull with the hands. Don't do it! *Let gravity do the work and focus on deep breath and relaxation.*

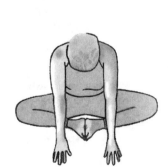

Day 3: Shoulders

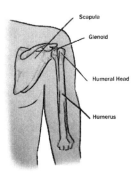

The shoulder is a complex joint with an equally complex group of muscles and connective tissues supporting it.

Tight shoulders are one of the most common complaints I hear from people of all walks of life, and the areas that need the most work are the muscles of the upper back such as the rhomboids, trapezius, and deltoids, to name a few.

In plain English, **to loosen up the shoulders, you need to loosen up the muscles of the upper back and arms** through highly-targeted stretches. In our normal lives, most of us rarely even lift our arms above our heads, much less stretch our shoulders, so it's no wonder that these poses can be so challenging at first.

SIGNS OF TIGHT SHOULDERS
- ✓ Hunched-forward posture
- ✓ Sore neck
- ✓ Poor backbends

WHO CARES ABOUT MY SHOULDERS?

Opening your shoulders opens up the front of your body and exposes your heart. Of all the areas we'll work on, improving the flexibility of your shoulders can be particularly liberating, both physically and emotionally.

Tight shoulders make you feel claustrophobic, stressed-out, and tense all day long. I say this because I used to have extremely tight shoulders, but I used these simple Gravity Poses to change that.

Here's the good news: once your shoulders open up, you'll be amazed at the freedom and strength you'll feel in your entire upper body. For athletic activities like tennis, golf, or basketball, people with open shoulders always outperform people who are stiff.

Day 3: Hangman

THE SETUP

1 – Lie on your belly with your head right up against the wall.

2 – Don't move your body forward or backward.

3 – Reach your arms up the wall with your hands wider than your shoulders.

4 – Spread your fingers, drop your head, and relax.

5 – Hold for 2-5 minutes.

6 – If your hands slip down, use your fingers to crawl your hands back up the wall.

 TIPS:

- This pose is <u>intense</u> and you really have to focus to stay calm.
- Allow your heart to melt between your shoulders.
- Let your head drop completely.
- Keep your arms straight, but as soft as possible.
- Decide <u>before</u> you start how long you're going to stay in this one... otherwise you'll come out too early.

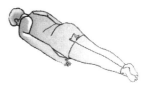

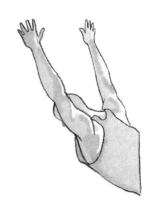

This pose is no joke. I used to shudder when I came out of it... I thought my top half was going to break off!

So take it slow!

Two minutes is usually a good starting point, but you can grow quickly with this pose. Most everyone should be able to do 3 minutes or more within 30 days. Normally, it's difficult to isolate the shoulder-restricting muscles of the upper back, but the Hangman gets right in there!

This pose alone took my backbends WAY deeper than I thought I'd ever go.

Day 3: Pretzel Arms

THE SETUP

1 – Lie on your belly.
2 – Using your right fingers, crawl your right hand as far to the LEFT as possible.

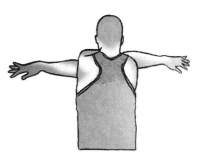

3 – Using your left fingers, crawl your left hand as far to the RIGHT as possible (over the top of the right arm).
4 – Spread your fingers.
5 – Drop your head and let the weight of your head rest on your arms.
6 – Soften your entire body and stay here for 3-5 minutes.
7 – Switch arms and repeat.

TIPS:
- This is awkward, so don't try to fix it—just accept it.
- Your head weight is important, so relax your neck and allow your chin to rest on your arms.
- Your body will want to tip to one side, so use as little energy as possible to stay in the middle.

This is perhaps the most awkward of all the Gravity Poses—but it's incredibly effective at isolating the muscles of the outer arm and upper back that can restrict shoulder mobility.

The first week you practice this, it's going to feel really weird, but the more you do it, the more you'll start to love it. Your shoulders can be so difficult to loosen up—and this pose makes a big difference fast.

Day 3: Wide Dog

THE SETUP

1 –   Step your feet about 1 – 1 ½ meters apart.

2 –   Bring your hands a little wider than your shoulders.

3 –   Spread your fingers wide.

4 –   Your hands should be closer to your feet than in a normal down dog you may have learned in yoga class.

5 –   Drop your head, look at your belly button, and relax.

6 –   Allow your body weight to sink completely into your shoulders.

7 –   Stay here for 3-5 minutes.

 TIPS:

- This is a different kind of down dog than you may have done before.
- Let your body go very soft, especially in the heart and chest area.
- Imagine your heart melting down as your shoulders soften in toward each other.
- You can bend your knees slightly if you feel a strain in the lower back.

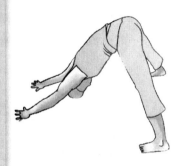

When my shoulders were really tight, I used to do this posture every morning for five minutes before I did anything else. After just 4 weeks, I'd made such big gains that I was suddenly able to jump through from down dog into a seated position without touching the ground.

As with all these poses, the key is to stay still, breathe deeply, and allow gravity to do the work naturally.

Day 4: Back

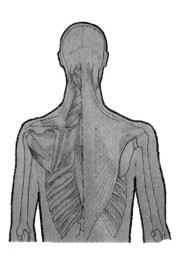

When people talk about stretching their back or spine, what they're actually talking about is stretching the muscles that support the spine through back bending exercises.

Since most people rarely (if ever) bend backwards in their normal, everyday lives, backbends are often VERY challenging, but also *very important for avoiding injury, relieving stress, and ensuring spinal strength and mobility.*

SIGNS OF A TIGHT BACK

   ✓ Hunched-forward posture
   ✓ Poor backbends
   ✓ Pain or strain, most-often in the lower back

WHY ARE BACKBENDS SO HARD?

In order to bend backwards, we need to open up the front of our body. This includes the muscles of the **abdomen**, the **intercostals**, the **shoulders**, and the **tops of the legs**. When compared with seated forward bends that do a great job of isolating the hamstring muscles; backbends are very gross stretches that involve a whole series of major muscle groups.

Together, all these tissues can really put up a fight against any sort of backward-bending movements you might be attempting.

So what do you do? You hold the poses longer, practice VERY carefully, breathe deeply—and give it some time! Progress in backbends **seems** slower, but because you're stretching so many different areas at once, every small gain is actually a huge gain in mobility for the entire front of your body.

Day 4: Lightning Bolt

THE SETUP

1 – Bring your knees together, feet apart.

2 – Sit down on the floor between your heels <u>or</u> on a folded up towel or pillow.

3 – If you can sit on the floor with no knee pain, you can lower yourself down onto your back one elbow at a time.

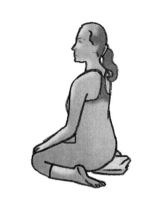

4 – If you feel any sharp, shooting knee pain, <u>do not</u> go down on your back, instead stay seated and back off a little.

5 – Either sitting up <u>or</u> lying down, hold for 2-5 minutes.

6 – Try to keep your knees close together if possible.

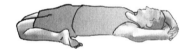

 TIPS:

- You <u>must</u> be careful with your knees here.
- If you feel pain, back off!
- Breathe deeply and allow your legs to completely relax.
- Don't force it; take it slowly.
- Come in and out cautiously.

There are a number of muscles on the tops of your legs that affect pelvic rotation, and since pelvic rotation has a huge impact on your ability to backbend, we need to loosen up our legs!

Two notable leg muscles are the psoas and iliacus which both start at the femur (leg bone). The iliacus inserts at the pelvic bowl while the psoas actually crosses the pelvis and connects to the lumbar spine.

What does this mean? Basically, if the tops of your legs are stiff, your pelvis can't tilt much; and if your pelvis can't tilt much, then all the pressure from back-bending goes right into your lower back—hence, the chronic back pain that so many people experience.

This pose alone can be more effective at opening your back than many of the common back-bending postures taught in yoga classes.

Day 4: Noodle

THE SETUP

1 – Use a chair or a stool with a cushion or pillow.

2 – Lie down carefully; extend your arms and legs.

3 – Relax your entire body and breathe.

4 – Hold for 4-5 minutes.

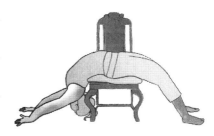

 TIPS:

- Many people are scared to release their head—don't be scared!
- Relax your head, neck, arms and legs completely.
- Don't worry if your hands and/or legs are not touching the floor.
- Be careful when you come up.

This is a very simple, passive way to open up the entire front of your body, freeing up your spine for greater mobility. *Avoid the temptation to force your back deeper or reach with your hands and feet.*

Noodle pose makes use of gravity to the fullest extent as your entire body is gently stretched. It's an excellent way to lengthen the tops of the legs, the intercostals (muscles between each rib), the abdomen, the shoulders, and the upper back. The best part is, you can do this pose anywhere, at any time—*just don't do it right after eating!*

Day 4: Shoulder Pow!

THE SETUP

1 –   Take any seated position.
2 –   Take your right arm straight up into the air.
3 –   Bend at the elbow, reach back and clasp your hands behind your back.
4 –   At first, it may not be possible to clasp hands, so use a small hand towel or belt.
5 –   Gently lean your head back into your arm, and relax.
6 –   Hold for 3-5 minutes.
7 –   Switch sides and repeat.

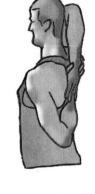

 TIPS:

- *You **must** hold onto something,* so if you can't reach your fingers yet, use a towel or belt—but make sure you hold something!
- The body has a tendency to curl forward here, so instead, sit up tall and gently lean your head back.

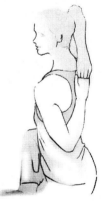

This intense pose will help you find space in your middle and upper back which is essential for safe back-bending. If your upper back is locked up, that means your lower back has to take all the pressure to compensate, which can lead to slipped or bulging discs and other complications.

This pose is very targeted so you'll progress very quickly. As you feel more space and opening, clasp your hands closer and closer, until eventually, you can grab wrists behind the back.

Day 5: Wrists, Twists & Ankles

B oth the wrists and ankles are part of a complex group of bones, joints, and muscles that are often stiff, sore, and tight from overuse or lack of use.

Lateral twising is another movement that we rarely do in our normal lives, so it's an essential part of any stretching regime that will help you avoid injury and build strength in the midsection.

SIGNS OF TIGHT WRISTS, TWISTS & ANKLES

✓ Pain or stiffness in the wrists or ankles
✓ Back pain
✓ Sore feet and hands
✓ Weak and bloated midsection

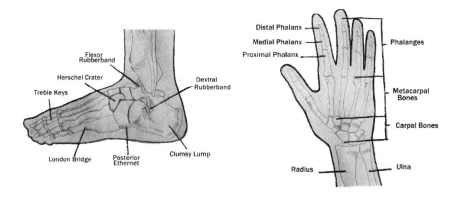

WHY BOTHER?

As we age, it's common for people to have curled-up hands from tight connective tissues or clenched feet from years of wearing small shoes. Without flexibility in our hands, wrists, feet, and ankles, simple tasks like writing and walking can become painful and cause soreness.

Twisting is also important because without lateral flexibility, simple activities like moving furniture or throwing a ball can cause massive muscle strains. ***Twisting also massages and aids in the detoxification of all the organs of digestion.***

Day 5: Reverse Dog

THE SETUP

1 – On your hands and knees, rotate your hands externally so that your middle fingers point toward your knees.

2 – Gently lean forward until you feel a big stretch in your wrists that extends up the forearms.

3 – If you feel comfortable here, you can lift up into down dog, with your hands in reverse—*but be careful!*

4 – Hold here either with knees on the ground or in reverse dog for 2-4 minutes.

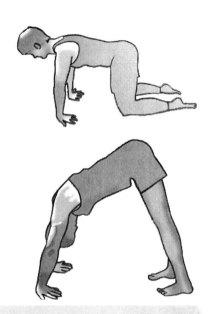

 TIPS:

- This can be really intense, so take it easy!
- If you feel sharp pain, back off immediately.
- Allow your head and neck to be heavy.
- Relax your body as much as possible.

It's important to know your limits, and in this pose, you'll find your limit very quickly! When you feel you're at your edge, stay still, practice deep breathing, and let the pose happen naturally.

This posture is highly targeted, which means you'll get results fast, but you also need to practice mindfully. If it's too intense to hold for long periods, another option is to practice this twice, each time holding for a minute or so.

Day 5: Twister

THE SETUP

1 –   Lie on your back.
2 –   Lift your legs into the air and bend your knees.
3 –   Cross your right leg over your left leg.
4 –   Try to 'double cross' your legs, if possible, so the right foot wraps around the left shin.
5 –   If you cannot double cross, it's okay.
6 –   Using your left hand, gently press your crossed legs toward the floor.
7 –   Stretch your right arm all the way straight out to the right.
8 –   Turn your head and look to the right.
9 –   Hold for 4-5 minutes.
10 – Switch sides and repeat.

TIPS:

- When you first begin, it's normal for both your knees and your extended arm to be up off the ground.
- Don't force your knees to the floor; just allow gravity to gently press down.
- Make sure your extended arm is all the way straight.
- Focus on complete exhales with each breath.

This gentle pose, when held for 4 or 5 minutes, will dramatically improve your lateral twisting flexibility. If at first you cannot double-cross your legs, just give it some time.

After a few weeks, most people are able to wrap at least their toes around the shin, which deepens the stretch and increases the benefits.

Day 5: Pins 'n Needles

THE SETUP

1 – Bring your knees together, tuck your toes under, and sit down on your heels.

2 – Bring your hands behind your back in a reverse prayer position.

3 – If reverse prayer is not possible, just grab your elbows behind your back.

4 – Sit down so the weight is heavy into your heels and toes.

5 – Gently press the hands closer together, press your elbows backwards, and keep the chin lifted.

6 – Hold for 2-5 minutes.

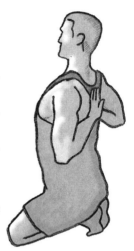

TIPS:

- You'll feel this in your toes and feet very intensely, very quickly—this is normal.
- If you experience any sharp, shooting pain in the knees—back off!
- Despite the fact that your toes <u>feel</u> like they're going to break off, they won't.
- Resist the urge to lean forward; instead, sit down onto the heels.
- Try to get your hands into a reverse prayer position (even an attempt will be beneficial), but if it's just not working, you can also grab your elbows behind your back.

This pose will make you want to wiggle and squirm more than anything. It's called Pins 'n Needles because that's what you'll feel in your feet, but fight the urge to move. You may feel like you want to scream while practicing Pins 'n Needles, but afterwards, your wrists, feet, and ankles will love you for it.

FREQUENT QUESTIONS

Many nutritional supplement companies like to keep their formulas and ingredients a secret, but at YOGABODY, we keep our entire operation completely transparent. We feel that the more you learn about us, the more you'll love YOGABODY and our practice aids.

YOGABODY is formulated by me, a yoga teacher, specifically for yoga and stretching students—and it REALLY works!

I'm very picky about what I put into my body, and I know you are too. Below are answers to some of the most commonly asked questions to help you better understand what it is you're taking.

EFFECTIVE: Does YOGABODY really work?

Absolutely, 100% guaranteed. YOGABODY is not some big pharmaceutical company trying to cash in on consumers' ignorance or hoping for the placebo effect to carry them to the bank. YOGABODY is formulated specifically for stretching students, and it makes practice easier. Period.

FLEXIBILITY: Will it make me more flexible?

There is no magic pill for flexibility, but YOGABODY Stretch has been shown to optimize flexibility, meaning that students often feel loose and limber—as though they've been practicing for 30 minutes or so—before they even begin class.

Because of this, students say their stretching exercises and yoga poses are more efficient with less time spent warming up and more time spent lengthening and stretching.

SAFE: Is YOGABODY safe?

YOGABODY Stretch is an all-natural, water-soluble supplement. This means that what your body doesn't need, you'll urinate out. It's not a medicine or drug; it's a whole food-based practice aid.

YOGABODY Stretch is made in an ultra-hygienic, FDA-inspected lab without the use of any flow agents (fillers) or additives. We're a small company and we know our suppliers personally.

I'm very picky about what I put into my body, and YOGABODY Stretch is micro-processed, ultra-pure, and passes my personal scrutiny with flying colors.

NOTE: *People with sulfur allergies or kidney disease should contact their doctor before use. Also if you're on medications or pregnant, seek professional advice.*

SPEED: How quickly does YOGABODY take effect?

In theory, YOGABODY Stretch should take a week or two to work. In reality, 90% of the participants in my case studies experienced benefits immediately—within an hour of the first dose.

Everyone's body is different, but yoga students seem to be particularly responsive to supplements, and YOGABODY Stretch in particular.

Commonly reported benefits include a loose, limber body, a feeling of lightness, decreased pain and soreness, increased energy and focus, curbed hunger, and strengthened digestion.

FORM: How is YOGABODY taken (liquid, capsule, powder, etc.)?

YOGABODY Stretch comes in 800 mg vegetarian (microcrystalline cellulose) capsules that are easy to swallow. If you don't like swallowing capsules, open them up, mix the powder with water, and drink quickly (it will taste quite bitter).

YOGA STUDENTS: Why do yoga students use YOGABODY?

YOGABODY Stretch is the only supplement formulated by a yoga teacher specifically for stretching and yoga students, and it REALLY does make practice easier. Consume with confidence.

DURATION: How long do the effects of YOGABODY last?

YOGABODY Stretch has both short and long-term effects. In the short term (4-6 hours), it's been shown to relieve inflammation, boost energy, and reduce soreness. In the long term, it's a potent source of vitamins, minerals, and anti-oxidants that help to heal and build muscle and connective tissues.

HOW MUCH/HOW OFTEN: How many capsules should I take?

If you're practicing stretching exercises regularly, start with two capsules twice per day and gradually increase to three capsules twice per day (6 per day total). 4-6 capsules is the ideal dosage for those with consistent practices. Less is fine, but if you take more, you'll just pee it out.

TOO MUCH: Is it possible to take too much?

If you take more than 4-6 capsules per day, you'll urinate out the excess. Taking large doses should be avoided since this will put unnecessary strain on your organs of elimination.

NON-ADDICTIVE: Is YOGABODY addictive?

Just like broccoli, YOGABODY Stretch is non-addictive. Like broccoli though, once you get into it, it's really nice to have around the house.

INGREDIENTS: What are the ingredients of YOGABODY [fleximine™]?

Each ingredient in YOGABODY Stretch is a superfood in and of itself, but the combination of these ingredients is what makes it so effective.

Here's what it contains:
- **MSM** (methylsulfonylmethane)
- **Triple Green Blend** (organic spirulina, organic chlorella, barley grass juice extract)
- **Ultra-Sorb Vit C** (ascorbic acid buffered with calcium ascorbate)
- **Trace Mineral Uptake Enhancers**

VEGETARIAN/VEGAN: Is YOGABODY vegetarian and/or vegan?

It's absolutely 100% vegetarian & vegan. Change your diet; change the world.

CHILDREN: Can children use YOGABODY?

This formula is designed for the needs of today's active stretching and yoga students. Children rarely fall into this category. YOGABODY Stretch is not harmful for children, but it's not appropriate or necessary.

STIMULANTS & PAINKILLERS: Does YOGABODY contain stimulants and/or painkillers?

No stimulants. No painkillers. No hocus pocus. Many students notice a boost in energy from YOGABODY, but not at all like the artificial, anxious energy boost of caffeine or other stimulants. It's believed that the energy boost comes from increased oxygen in the blood from the blast of nutrients that YOGABODY Stretch delivers in ideal ratios.

Avoid taking at least 3 hours before bedtime as it may inhibit sleep.

SIDE-EFFECTS: Does YOGABODY have any side-effects?

YOGABODY Stretch is an all-natural, water-soluble supplement. Very rarely (less than 1% of case study participants), users experience an upset stomach which can easily be avoided by decreasing the dosage or taking the capsules with food until your body adjusts.

NOTE: *People with sulfur allergies or kidney disease should contact their doctor before use. Also if you're on medications or pregnant, seek professional advice.*

NATURAL/ORGANIC: Is YOGABODY all-natural and/or organic?

My business is an extension of my life. I'm a vegan, an organic farm supporter, and an optimistic environmentalist—so whenever possible, we buy organic or organically-grown ingredients. If it's not natural, we don't use it.

COST: Why is YOGABODY so inexpensive?

I buy in bulk directly from the source, and I keep my operational costs as low as possible. In this way, I'm able to offer huge bottles (180 capsules as opposed to the industry standard of 90) of what is essentially a 6-in-1 supplement at a cost lower than most single-ingredient supplements.

GIRL ON THE BOTTLE: Who is the girl on the bottle?

The girl on the bottle is a friend and yoga teacher named Mon Napassawan. She teaches at Absolute Yoga in Thailand and has a beautiful practice.

100% GUARANTEE: What is the YOGABODY guarantee?

YOGABODY ingredients have proven effective both by the medical community and in case studies of yoga students and teachers. I use it every day. It REALLY works, and I stand behind all purchases 100% with a 365-day, unconditional guarantee. No questions. No fine print.

ABOUT THE AUTHOR

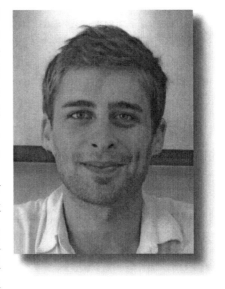

Yoga teacher and nutritional coach, Lucas Rockwood, studied raw food nutrition with Gabriel Cousens M.D. at The Tree of Life in Patagonia, AZ, and later went on to run Caravan of Dreams, New York City's long-standing, iconic vegetarian restaurant.

First in Los Angeles and New York City, then later in Bangkok and Hong Kong, Lucas studied, taught, and experimented extensively with yoga and nutrition until he found certain principles and practices that are simple, effective, and universally applicable. His yoga asana teachers include Paul Dallaghan, Alex Medin, and Sri K. Pattabhi Jois.

"With a regular yoga practice, a plant-based diet, and specific nutritional supplements, it's possible to radically change your state of health in a matter of months," says Lucas, who himself lost 41 lbs. and increased his flexibility tenfold using a program he now calls The YOGABODY Revolution.

Lucas says, *"Naturally, we're lean, limber, and healthy. Yoga, a proper diet, and superfood supplements can help you return to that natural state—quickly!"*

In 2006, Lucas co-founded **Absolute Yoga & The Love Kitchen**, a yoga studio and health food restaurant on Koh Samui island in Thailand where he continues to host yoga courses and certification trainings throughout the year.

Lucas also conducts private nutritional coaching (via telephone) on an application-only basis to serious students interested in dramatically changing their lifestyle. To learn more about Lucas and his work, please visit any of his websites:

YOGABODY – Flexibility training materials, nutritional supplements, and online community *www.YogaBodyNaturals.com*

YOGA PROTEIN – The ultimate sprouted brown rice protein supplement for busy people who want to stay strong and lean *www.YogaProtein.com*

THE YOGA TRAPEZE – Back pain gone in 7 minutes... the ultimate spine-strength and flexibility tool that's a ton of fun *www.TheYogaTrapeze.com*

THE BUSINESS OF TEACHING YOGA – Learn how to earn a great living teaching yoga anywhere in the world *www.MyYogaBusiness.com*

YOGA COURSES & TEACHER TRAININGS – Beautiful Thailand island yoga center where Lucas hosts courses throughout the year *www.AbsoluteYogaSamui.com*

HOT YOGA HOME STUDY COURSE – Lucas' friend Gabrielle in Australia has put together an amazing course *www.HotYogaGuru.com*

For event bookings, teaching engagements, product inquires, and consulting, please contact Lucas' office directly:

Lucas Rockwood   310.878.4829 (USA)
                                lucas@yogabodynaturals.com

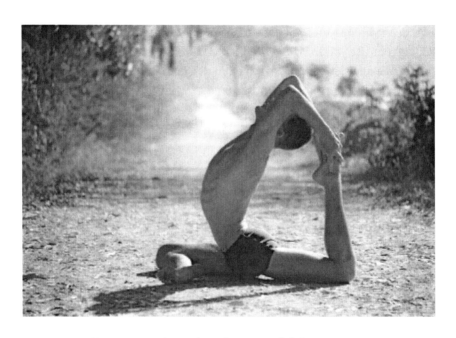

"Yoga exists in the world because
everything is linked"
~ *T.K.V. Desikachar*

FREE YOGA RESOURCES

Visit: www.YogaBodyNaturals.com to Claim Your Gifts!

Dear Yoga Student,

If you enjoyed this book and want to learn more ways to improve your practice at home—or even how to become a yoga teacher yourself— then I'd like to invite you to visit my YOGABODY website where you can sign up for my free newsletter and join our extended community that now includes over 10,000 students in 31 countries (and growing).

Here's what you'll find at **www.YogaBodyNaturals.com:**

- Free stretching tips, tricks & practices
- Free videos & articles
- Free yoga wallpapers (for your computer)
- Free yoga iPhone Applications
- Free audio classes (both on CD or streaming .mp3)
- My powerful superfood supplements and practice tools catalog

If you get excited about personal transformation and radical health unleashed by yoga practice and lifestyle choices—or if you're just curious to see what this YOGABODY community is all about—then visit me and the gang online or drop me an email anytime.

Yoga is my passion in life, and I want to thank you for giving me this opportunity to share what I've learned with you. I hope to see you in class or in a workshop or retreat very soon... until then, keep practicing and enjoy the ride!

Stay bendy,

Lucas Rockwood
YOGABODY Naturals LLC
Find Me Here: **www.YogaBodyNaturals.com**

CPSIA information can be obtained
at www.ICGtesting.com
Printed in the USA
FSOW02n1336230215
5303FS